Type 1 Diabetes

The Resolution

By Cinnamon Quinones-Gilmore

These statements have not been evaluated by the FDA. This product is not intended to diagnose, treat, cure, or prevent any disease

Introduction

Type 1 Diabetes is often a disorder that gets little conversation because it is said to be rare and "incurable". Type 1 Diabetes isn't as common as Type 2 Diabetes. As a matter of fact, there are tons of people who aren't aware that they have Type 1 Diabetes. This disorder is identified as an autoimmune disease that affects the endocrine system. It is also identified with hyperthyroidism and Graves' disease in some people.

There are pharmaceutical medications that help to mask some of the symptoms of Type 1 Diabetes. Medications such as Vasopressin, Insulin, and more. No one wants to live everyday of their lives taking medications that almost always have undesirable side effects.

What about natural remedies for Type 1 Diabetes? Not everyone is aware that certain herbs exist that can help to reverse Type 1 Diabetes along with a better lifestyle. This book will give you information that could only improve your health and help you to potentially reverse this disorder.

Index

<u>What is Type 1 Diabetes?</u>

Type 1 Diabetes (T1D) happens when the body starts to attack itself via the endocrine system, thus making it an autoimmune disease. T1D also occurs when the pancreas doesn't create nor produce enough insulin via Islet Langerhans (insulin producing tissue). Insulin is a hormone produced by the cells of the pancreas. The inability of the pancreas to create these cells/hormones is the main cause of T1D.

The endocrine system is responsible for the pancreas, thyroid, ovaries, testes, adrenal, pineal gland, pituitary gland, and the hypothalamus gland.

<u>The Pancreas:</u> The pancreas is the gland that is responsible for both the endocrine and exocrine systems as well as how they function. The endocrine system produces hormones called glucagon and insulin while the exocrine system produces digestive enzymes. The pancreas is seated behind the stomach.

<u>The Thyroid:</u> The thyroid is responsible for producing thyroid hormones that balances the body's metabolism. The thyroid manages bone growth as well as how the nervous system develops in children. The thyroid gland is also responsible for metabolism, digestion, heart rate, muscle health, and blood pressure.

There are also parathyroid glands that release hormones that manages the calcium levels and iron levels. The thyroid is a butterfly shaped gland located at the base of the neck.

<u>The Reproductive Glands:</u> The reproductive glands are the main source of sex hormones via testes and ovaries. These glands regulate testosterone and estrogen levels. It also affects development of sperm and eggs.

<u>The Pineal Gland:</u> The pineal gland is located core of the brain. This gland is responsible for secreting melatonin and helps to manage the wake-sleep cycle.

<u>Adrenal Glands:</u> These are two glands located at the top of the kidneys. One of the adrenal glands is called the outer part (corticosteroids) or

The adrenal cortex. This helps balance the salt and water in the body, helps the immune system, and manages sexual functions. The second gland called the inner part (catecholamine) or the adrenal medulla helps the body to fight both emotional and physical stress by managing the blood pressure and heart rate.

Hypothalamus Gland: This gland is located via the central part of the brain. The hypothalamus gland balances metabolism and body temperature. This gland also secretes hormones via the pituitary gland which can either stimulate or suppress the cells.

Pituitary Glands: This gland is located near the base of the brain. It is so small that it is just a tad bit smaller than a pea. The pituitary gland has two parts- The anterior lobe and posterior lobe.

The anterior lobe contains different hormones, one is called ACTH (Adrenocorticotropin hormone) that stimulates the adrenal gland in order to produce enough steroid hormones. The ACTH also controls the growth hormones via muscle, tissue, bone mass, and body fat.

LH (Luteinizing Hormone) and FSH (Follicle Stimulating Hormone)
stimulates the production and function of the sex steroids via estrogen
and progesterone in females and testosterone in males. Prolactin is a
hormone that regulates milk production in a female who is lactating.

The posterior lobe controls vasopressin which is the antidiuretic
hormone that controls the water that is excreted out of the body via the
kidneys. The posterior lobe also controls Oxytocin which helps the
uterus to contract during childbirth as well as stimulates the production
of milk.

Disorders of the endocrine such as T1D are common metabolic disorders
in children and adolescents. There are even some cases where children
have developed benign brain tumors as a result. Some children even
have trouble controlling their bladders because of glands such as the
pituitary which controls the vasopressin.

Symptoms of T1D are blurred vision, unexplained weight loss, frequent urination, nausea, dry skin, increased hunger & thirst, hair loss, fast heart rate, and trouble focusing. T1D is also known as water diabetes, diabetes insipidus, and brittle diabetes.

 We will break down the certain symptoms or other diseases of T1D as they may or may not be associated with the disease as a whole. Treating symptoms of T1D may ultimately lead to overall reversal of the disorder. Each part of the endocrine system will need to be addressed for desired results.

- Hyperthyroidism is when the thyroid produces too much of its hormones. Because of the overproduction, the body speeds up its metabolism resulting in unwanted weight loss, irregular and/or rapid heartbeat, anxiety attacks, irritability, and in some cases insomnia.
- Polyuria or Diuresis is a disorder that causes frequent urination and causes abnormally large volumes of urine to be excreted. This can be associated with the weight loss of T1D and Hyperthyroidism.

- Hyperglycemia is when a person's glucose level is too high, also known as high blood sugar. This can be linked to the increased hunger and dehydration symptoms of T1D. Although that person is eating and drinking enough, their bodies cannot properly absorb minerals and hold water also resulting in weight loss, dehydration, and malnourishment. This is also due to the increased or high metabolism via the overactive thyroid or hyperthyroidism.

- Women who have hyperthyroidism may have trouble producing enough milk for their babies. The pituitary and thyroid glands are responsible for stimulating the hormones to produce enough milk. But when the mother can't store an adequate amount of minerals and water for her own body it will be hard for her to produce more milk.

- Tachycardia is the term for rapid heart rate. This is the most common symptom of T1D. An accelerated heart rate means that there is not enough blood flowing to the heart. This can ultimately lead to high blood pressure. Some people have even reported blacking out or losing their vision briefly when they are experiencing a rapid heart rate with T1D.

- (RLS) Restless Leg Syndrome is a disorder that occurs while someone is sleeping or at rest. This involves a pain, tingling, crawling or numbing sensation on the legs while asleep. This is the result of high blood pressure, kidney issues, and overactive thyroid.

- Hair loss is another common symptom associated with T1D and hyperthyroidism. These disorders can cause the hair to thin, become brittle, and easily fall out. The thyroid hormones T3 (Triiodothyronine, most active) and T4 (Thyroxine) is overproduced when it conjoins with iodine. This causes the hair to fall out.

<u>Herbal Remedies vs Pharmaceutical Remedies</u>

<u>*Please be cautious of taking herbs while consuming pharmaceutical medication. Ask your doctors before use and if pregnant or nursing*</u>

There are pharmaceuticals that are prescription only that will help to mask the symptoms of T1D or keep it at bay to keep the body from attacking itself via the endocrine system. However, pharmaceuticals aren't meant to be taken long term because of the side effects that most people experience. It is always safer to take more natural alternatives.

There are some antithyroid medication that relieves symptoms and prevents the thyroid from excessively produce hormones.

- Vasopressin occurs naturally in our bodies, but it is also created synthetically. Vasopressin is an ADH (antidiuretic hormone). When this hormone isn't created enough to be released it can lead to excessive water loss. Vasopressin is available via prescription to help control an overactive bladder.

- Desmopressin is a synthetic type of vasopressin. The most common brand is DDAVP (desamino-cys-d-arg- vasopressin). It works the same way as the prescription vasopressin. Although the

- desmopressin is available in tablets it is commonly used as a nasal spray.

- Arginine isn't a mineral but instead an amino acid which is created through biosynthesis. It isn't necessarily made as a pharmaceutical, but it doesn't present itself in nature either. Getting Arginine can only be done via what you put into your body. You can take it as a vitamin or food such as meats. Arginine is said to control the enzyme structure and function, maintains heart health, and it is commonly used for erectile dysfunction.

- Radioactive Iodine (I-131) is most commonly used in the U.S as an antithyroid treatment. The I-131 is taken by mouth and absorbed through the bloodstream to delay or kill the cells of the thyroid gland. There are many side effects after taking this treatment such as dry mouth, dry eyes, nausea, swelling of the neck, and swelling of the salivary glands.

- There are more natural remedies to help treat T1D. The herbalist Dr. Sebi has mentioned Brittle Diabetes in one of his lectures. Dr. Sebi was an herbalist from Honduras who has claimed to have cured people from many illnesses including T1D. His methodology was the alkaline diet and the removal of mucus to allow the body to heal itself.

"Now, when your bones are brittle you need calcium, right? But when the Islet of Langerhans are all obstructed, what they need now? Chromium. Because the pancreas is Chromium,"- Dr. Sebi. There are foods and herbs that are alkaline specified that could help the symptoms and overall resolution of T1D. The tomato, lettuce, and kale are high in chromium. There are herbs that Dr. Sebi has used to treat Diabetes that are also high in chromium such as Nettle, Blue Vervain, Wild Yam, Bugleweed, Cascara Sagrada, Horsetail, Valerian, but other alkaline herbs will be listed. Not only do these herbs have chromium to help nourish the pancreas but they also aid the endocrine system:

- Cascara Sagrada (*Rhamnus Purshiana*)- This herb stimulates the secretions in the liver, pancreas, and gallbladder and it treats severe cases of constipation. Cascara also treats hemorrhoids, anorexia, bloating, and dyspepsia. It helps stools to move smoothly and it also regulates hormones that assists the pancreas to manage insulin, blood sugar and glucagon.

- Valerian (*Valeriana Officianalis*)- This herb is a sedative and relieves stress. It treats insomnia, anxiety, and nervousness. Valerian is also said to have antidiuretic hormones.

- Bugleweed (*Lycopus Virginicus*)- This herb is able to block TSH (thyroid-stimulating hormone) production. Bugleweed lowers levels of thyroid hormones and regulates the body's heartbeat. It helps to treat Graves' disease, anxiety, heavy menstruation, and breast pains.

- Stinging Nettle (*Urtica Diocia*)- Helps to treat urination problems such as urinary tract infections, frequent urination, nighttime urination, and difficulty passing urine. Nettle helps to lower blood pressure and sugar. It treats alopecia, anemia, poor circulation, heart problems, rashes, hay fever, and prostate diseases.

- Wild Yam (*Dioscorea Villosa*)- Helps to balance estrogen and other reproductive hormones. Wild Yam helps the body to produce energy and to treat menopause. It aids in vaginal dryness, weak bones and arthritis. It has even been noted to cause slight breast enlargement.

- Rosemary (*Rosmarinus Officinalis*)- Rosemary aids in healthy blood pressure, kidney problems, diabetes, baldness, chest pain, heartburn, flatulence, and decreases the amount of protein in the urine. Rosemary has also been shown to regulate thyroid functions.

- Thyme (*Thymus Vulgaris*)- In my opinion, Thyme doesn't get enough credit for what it really does. A lot of people use it as a garnish, but it is actually a multipurpose herb. Thyme can relieve sore throats, bronchitis, and other respiratory issues, along with skin issues, teeth cleaning, and bad breath. It is also said to cleanse and disinfect the urine ridding it of harmful "protein" that could cause urinary tract infections.

- Blue Vervain (*Verbana Hastata*)- Dr. Sebi noted the Blue Vervain as being on of his favorite herbs. Blue Vervain can assist with regulating the central nervous system as well as the reproductive system. It is high in zinc, phosphorus, and iron fluorine which can play a major role in immunity, blood health, and heart health. Blue Vervain also helps the female body to produce the hormone prolactin, when she is nursing, thus promoting milk production. This herb also helps to regulate metabolic disorders.

- Horsetail (*Equistum Arvense*)- Helps to treat an overactive bladder associated with diabetes. Horsetail also aids in respiratory health such as sinusitis, bronchitis, blocked nasal passages, congestion, as well as the cold and flu. Horsetail is most reputable for hair, skin, and nail health. It also aids in wound healing.

<u>Other Herbs That Show Promising Results</u>

The herbs that will be listed on this chapter are not alkaline approved. Neither do we know for sure if some of them are actually alkaline approved because of Dr. Sebi's untimely death in 2016. He provided a list of beneficial herbs and foods in his nutritional guide, however, there may have been some herbs that he may have approved but not noted.

There has been research about some herbs that show promising results when it comes to relieving symptoms of T1D:

- Anise (*Pimpinella Anisum*)- Anise oil has been noted to have antidiuretic effects as it reduces the volume of urine that is produced. Anise decreases bloating, cough, asthma, scabies, and lice.

- Gumby Gumby (*Pittosporum Angustifolium*)- Also known as Native Apricot and Butter bush, Gumby Gumby is a plant native to Australia. Gumby Gumby is known as the indigenous plant that helps detoxes the body and regulates the cardiovascular system.

Gumby Gumby also helps to treat cancer, fatigue, and depression. It is also a galactagogue meaning it stimulates the prolactin hormones to increase milk supply.

- Sumach (*Rhus Aromatica*)- This is a plant that helps to slow down fluid loss from any area of the body especially the kidneys. It also strengthens the kidneys and manages blood sugar levels. Sumach can also help with eyesight issues.

- Pumpkin Seed (*Cucurbita Pepo*)- Pumpkin seeds are known for ridding the body of parasites. Pumpkin seed has shown affects of decreasing frequent urination as well as kidney health. It improves insulin regulation and boosts testosterone in men.

- Lemon Balm (*Melissa Officinalis*)- Lemon Balm is quite popular for treating anxiety and depression. It is said to reduce thyroid hormone levels and relieves menstrual cramps. Lemon Balm can also be used for respiratory issues such as sinuses and allergies.

- Motherwort (*Leonurus Cardiaca*)- Motherwort is a plant that calms an overactive thyroid along with most of its symptoms such as fatigue, irregular heartbeat, a decrease in sex hormones, and nervousness. It can also aid in flatulence.

As I have noted before, although these herbs are not alkaline (some are still up for debate such as the Gumby Gumby), they have shown promising results for symptom relief of T1D.

<u>Case Studies</u>

As a person who is currently battling hyperthyroidism and as an active herbalist, I have decided to try some of these herbs for myself. Keep in mind that I am currently nursing a 6-month-old baby, thus that restricts me from consuming herbs such as Bugleweed, Horsetail, Thyme (in large doses) Wild Yam, Rosemary (in large doses), and Cascara Sagrada. However, I have conducted case studies on Valerian, Rosemary (in moderation), Blue Vervain, Stinging Nettle and Pumpkin Seed Oil.

Ask your doctor or practitioner if pregnant or lactating before consuming herbs

Having the symptoms of hyperthyroidism such as frequent urination, weight loss, irregular heartbeat, insomnia, blurred vision (since childhood), fatigue, trouble with focusing, hair loss, and dry skin I was very adamant on trying to improve my health.

- Valerian Case Study- I have always been a fan of Valerian. It eases your anxiety and can even help you get some rest. There was one time where I had taken two cups and fell asleep easily. Valerian is said to possibly have an antidiuretic affect. Please do not consume

Valerian if taking diuretics. For this particular case study, I had

consumed Valerian 5 days in a row. Along with decreasing my

anxiety and stress almost immediately, I had noticed that I didn't

take my usual frequent trips during the night to the bathroom. Thus

relieving me of the hyperthyroid symptom of frequent urination.

Valerian had also helped extremely with my insomnia. I took about

2 -3 cups daily.

- Blue Vervain is another herb that I have tried in its dried form, 600

  mg. I've consumed Blue Vervain for 5 days consecutively and

  noticed in increase in milk production. Also, my baby was in a

  calmer mood and crying less after a breastfeeding session. I've

  also noticed that the herb made me a bit lightheaded with no

  anxiety. Although I did see some improve with the Blue Vervain it

  is best to be used fresh. Dr. Sebi noted that this herb only lasted 6

  months in its dried form and you will experience the effects of

  Blue Vervain at its strongest while it is fresh. Unfortunately, it is

  only available fresh during the springtime.

- Stinging Nettle was an herb that I had also used for five days, about 1200 mg in a tincture. Nettle has been one my most favored herbs prior to this case study so overall, I am no stranger to its benefits. My heart rate wasn't high, my hair stopped shedding frequently and I even noticed my skin was less dry.
- Pumpkin seed is not approved to be alkaline but for the sake of this case study I gave it a try. I took one 2000 mg pill of pumpkin seed oil and noticed that I wasn't running to the bathroom throughout the day for frequent urination. However, I did notice a mild break out with my skin as well as bloating.

I've also noticed that a couple of food sources gave me relief of the hyperthyroidism symptoms. Prickly Pears (Cactus Fruit) and fresh squeezed blueberry juice. The prickly pear is the fruit of the Nopal cactus which has amazing benefits. It is very high in calcium and magnesium needed for both bone and brain health. Since the central nervous system is affected by hyperthyroidism and/or T1D it made sense to consume a large amount.

I took the pleasure in making eleven of the prickly pears and made fresh juice out of it with the prickly pear and spring water being the only ingredients. I drank an entire pitcher within a matter of 2 days and noticed many changes. My mood was very calm and I even had a lucid dream where my dreams were extremely vivid. I even woke up without congestion. Also, I noticed no body odor within the two-day span. My urine was very clear also. Prickly pear also is known to regulate the enzymes in your digestive system.

I did the same for blueberries. I made blueberry juice from 8 oz worth of blueberries and the only other ingredient was water. I made a pitcher's worth and noticed changes with my brain. After playing helicopter with my kids by spinning around in the kitchen, I started to have moderate nausea. My intent was to drink some ginger root tea, but I was too lazy to make it. My mouth was dry and I wanted something cold to drink so I drank a cup of my blueberry juice. My nausea went away instantly, and I had a burst of energy.

<u>Find the Match</u>

While doing research on T1D and the herbs that could possibly

hold the resolution for its overall presence I created a list that

connects the dots between the symptoms of T1D and the herbs that

can possibly reverse it.

- Pituitary Gland- Horsetail, Blue Vervain, Wild Yam, Valerian and

Nettle.

- Hypothalamus Gland- Bugleweed and BlueVervain.

- Adrenal Gland- Bugleweed, Blue Vervain, and Rosemary

- Pineal Gland- Valerian, Blue Vervain, and Nopal/Cactus fruit.

- Reproductive Glands- Bugleweed, Wild Yam, and Blue Vervain.

- Thyroid Gland- Bugleweed, Blue Vervain, Rosemary, Thyme,

Nettle.

- Pancreas- Cascara Sagrada, Nopal/Cactus fruit, and Rosemary.

Please refer to Chapter 1 to identify each function of the endocrine

system and keep in mind these herbs that benefit each gland the

most.

References:

- M. Schlumberger, M. Brose, R. Elisei, S. Leboulleux, and M. Luster. *Definition and management of radioactive iodine-refractory differentiated thyroid cancer.* The Lancet Diabetes & Endocrinology 2(5) 356-358, 2014.

- J.F. Goodwin, A.G. Macgregor, H. Miller, E.J. Wayne. *The use of radioactive iodine in the assessment of thyroid function.* QJM: An International Journal of Medicine 20(3), 353-387, 1951.

- T.A. Treschan (M.D.), J. Peters (M.D.). *The Vasopressin System: Physiology & Clinical Strategies.* Anesthesiology 9 2006, Vol 1. 105, 599-612. Doi: https://doi.org/

- S.I. Kreydiyyeh, J. Usta, S. Markossian, & S. Dagher, S. *Anise seed oil increases glucose absorption and reduces urine output in rat.* Life Sci 12-19-2003; 74(5): 663-673.

- Jacob P. Veenstra & Jeremy J. Johnson. *Oregano (Origanum Vulgare) extract for food preservation and improvement in gastro-intestinal health.* Int J. Nutr. Author manuscript; available in PM (2019 May 9. Published in final edited form as: Int J Nutr.2019; 3(4): 43-52. Doi: 10.14302/issn.2379-7835. Ijn-19-2703.

- Monica Damle. *Glycyrrhiza glabra (Liquorice) a potent medicinal herb.* International Journal of Herbal Medicine 2014; 2(2): 132-136. ISSN: 2321-2187.

- W. Curt LaFrance, Jr., M.D., Edward C. Lauterbach, M.D., C. Edward Coffey, M.D., Stephen P. Salloway, M.D., M.S., Daniel I. Kaufer, M.D., Alison Reeve, M.D. *The Use of Herbal Alternative Medicines in Neuropsychiatry.* A Report of the ANPA Committee on Research. J Neuropsychiatry Clin. Neuroset 12.2, Spring 2020.

- Leo T. Samuels, Nicholas W. Fugo. *The Antidiuretic Action of Yohimbine.* Endocrinology, Volume 34, Issue 3, 1 March 1944, Pages 143-148. Https://doi.org/10.1210/endo-34-3-143.

- Tania Shiminski-Maher, RN, MS, CPNP, CNRN July 1st, 1991. *Diabetes Insipidus & Syndrome of Inappropriate Secretion of Antidiuretic Hormone on Children with Midline Suprasellar Brain Tumor.* Journal of Pediatric Oncology Nursing.

- Nasim Mavahed, Hosein Zaeri, Maryam Razzaghy Azar. *The effect of urtica dioica extract on glycemic control of patients with Type 1 diabetes: a randomized, double-blind clinical trial.* Journal of Diabetes, Metabolic Disorders and Control: Volume 6 Issue 2-2019. Department of Pediatrics Golestan University of Medical Sciences, Iran. Received: March 08, 2019. Published: April 03, 2019.

- *Botanical Medicine for Thyroid Regulation.* Clinical Botanical Medicine Second Edition. Published: 23 May 2009.

- Solomon Habtemariam. *The Therapeutic Potential of Rosemary (Rosmarinus Officinalis) Diterpenes for Alzheimer's Disease.* Evid Based Complement Alternat Med. 2016. 2680409. Published online 2016 Ja 28. Doi:10.1155/2016/2680409.

- Eric Yarnell, N.D., R.H. (A.H.G) Kathy Abascal, J.D., R.H. (A.H.G). *Botanical Medicine for Thyroid Regulation.* Alternative & Complementary Therapies, Vol. 12, No. 3. Published Online: 12 Jun 2006 https://doi.org/10.10/act.2006.12.107.

- Leo Emmanuel Bunag, John Anthony Domantay 2016. *Thyrosuppressive Activity of Rosemary (Rosmarinus Officinalis) Leaves on experimentally-induced hyperthyroidism in male Sprague Dawley rats.* Itceprints.slu.edu.ph.

- Hebert, S.L., and Nair, K.S. (2010). Clinical Nutrition (Edinburgh, Scotland). 29(1), 13-17. Doi:10.1016/j.clnu.2009.09.001.

Cinnamon Quinones-Gilmore is an herbalist and wellness coach. She has received her credentials from the American College of Healthcare Sciences in Portland, OR with her AAS in Complementary Alternative Medicine with a focus in Herbal Medicine. Gilmore is also an educator in the Alkaline diet that the late Dr. Sebi promoted and encouraged amongst people who were suffering from incurable diseases.

Gilmore was born and raised in Cleveland, OH and is practicing herbal case studies there currently. She greatly believes that with the change of lifestyle and diet, anyone can achieve health. Gilmore has helped people overcome high blood pressure, hair loss, infertility, impotency, anemia, and many more reversals to come in the future. She hopes that her books will be a reference and guide to overcoming disease and bad eating habits.

Stay blessed!